I0465223

THE POSITIVE DIRECTION MODEL: OPIOID USE & PREGNANCY

First Edition

DAVINA MOSS-KING, PHD.

authorHOUSE®

AuthorHouse™
1663 Liberty Drive
Bloomington, IN 47403
www.authorhouse.com
Phone: 1 (800) 839-8640

© 2017 Davina Moss-King, PhD. All rights reserved.

No part of this book may be reproduced, stored in a retrieval system, or
transmitted by any means without the written permission of the author.

Published by AuthorHouse 03/15/2017

ISBN: 978-1-5246-6905-8 (sc)
ISBN: 978-1-5246-6904-1 (e)

Library of Congress Control Number: 2017901141

Print information available on the last page.

Any people depicted in stock imagery provided by Thinkstock are models,
and such images are being used for illustrative purposes only.
Certain stock imagery © Thinkstock.

This book is printed on acid-free paper.

Because of the dynamic nature of the Internet, any web addresses or links contained in
this book may have changed since publication and may no longer be valid. The views
expressed in this work are solely those of the author and do not necessarily reflect the
views of the publisher, and the publisher hereby disclaims any responsibility for them.

CONTENTS

DEDICATION

This book is dedicated to the women making lifestyle changes for the health and well- being of their infants. This book is also dedicated to the nurses and neonatologists that care for the infants in the Neonatal Intensive Care Unit that are diagnosed with Neonatal Abstinence Syndrome.

The Obstetrician / Gynecologists, Opioid maintenance Therapy providers, Behavioral Health Specialists, Substance Use Disorder Counselors along with the navigators that assist women through their journey.

A special thank you is extended to my beautiful daughters Nia and Naima, my husband Darryl; my parents Jerrell Moss and Genevieve Moss along with close friends and family members for their continued support.

ABOUT THE AUTHOR

Davina A. Moss-King, Ph.D., CRC, NCC, CASAC has been a substance abuse counselor for 25+ years. Dr. Moss-King is a Certified Rehabilitation Counselor, National Certified Counselor as well as a Credentialed Alcohol and Substance Abuse counselor in New York State. Dr. Moss-King received her doctorate in Counselor Education with honors in 2005 from the State University of New York at Buffalo. Her world acclaimed dissertation "Unresolved Grief and Loss Issues Related to Substance Abuse" was published as a book "Unresolved Grief and Loss Issues Related to Heroin Recovery," in 2009. Dr. Moss-King's research interest is opioid disorders and Neonatal Abstinence Syndrome which has evolved to writing an international accredited on-line course "Opioid Dependence during Pregnancy" (2015, 2017) from NetCE and World Continuing Education Alliance, along with an article entitled Neonatal Abstinence Syndrome – the Negative Effects On Our Future" (2015). Dr. Moss-King authored the chapter, "Individual Treatment," in the textbook *Substance Abuse and Treatment* 5th and 6th Editions (2013, 2017) and a chapter entitled "Addiction Psychology" for Bridgepoint College (2016).

Dr. Moss-King is an adjunct professor at Canisius College's Counselor Education and Human Services Department, Buffalo, NY.

Dr. Moss-King is the founder and President of Positive Direction and Associates, Inc.: consulting / counseling company that provides educational seminars focusing on opioid use disorders, women's health and rebuilding families.

Dr. Moss-King is a member of the American Psychological Association and the National Association of Neonatal Therapists.

CHAPTER 1

INTRODUCTION

The National Survey on Drug Use and Health statistics in their 2014 research stated that an estimated 225,000 infants are exposed to illicit substances each year and the numbers are increasing. Approximately 60-94% of neonates exposed to opioids during pregnancy will exhibit symptoms of Neonatal Abstinence Syndrome (NAS). NAS are a group of withdrawal symptoms experienced by the infant after birth affecting the autonomic, gastrointestinal and neurological systems. Statistics have shown that every 25 minutes an infant is exposed to opioids and experiences NAS after birth. In 2014 the annual health care cost for caring for NAS infants was 1.5 billion and was part of the hospital stay for infants in the Neonatal Intensive Care Unit (NICU) for 16 days or more. The cost for infants staying in the hospital past the average stay is approximately $66,700 as opposed to the cost for an infant born without NAS is $3000.00. These statistics are alarming and has caused an epidemic nationally and is having a negative effect on our future generations.

According to SAMHSA (2014), there have been 4.6 million women ages 18 and up that have misused prescription drugs within the reporting year 2013-2014. The misuse of the opioids has created a disenfranchised group of women in the areas of stigma, being judged by others, and this leads to women not obtaining the necessary treatment that is needed to begin recovery. The lack of necessary treatment can lead to a fear of reaching out for assistance for detoxification and or rehabilitation and in the event the woman is pregnant the lack of pre-natal care is harmful to the woman and her unborn infant. If the woman were to be given education early there will be an increase of self-awareness and collaboration of health care providers to create a healthy environment for the woman, her family and the infant. The Positive Direction Matrix (figure 1) is an illustration of the importance of educating the woman during her pregnancy and all of the components that are involved.

The Positive Direction Matrix

Health (Sobriety)	The woman will receive education regarding the need for sobriety and the negative effects on the fetus if the woman continues drugs and / or alcohol. Psycho-educational group work is an option to discuss the importance of nutrition and coping mechanisms to continue sobriety. This part of the matrix can be administered by a substance use disorder therapist along with other resources regarding health this is vital.
Family (Living Supports)	The woman will identify the persons that will be supportive during and after the pregnancy. At this point the woman will also discuss her place of residence and identifying if the residence is safe environment for her and the baby. During this time it is vital for the woman to learn from a navigator the supports that are needed and mostly, how the support(s) will be implemented and by whom.

Mental Health	The woman will be educated on the importance of mental health stability pre-natal and post-natal. The education will include but is not limited to symptoms of depression pre-natal and depression post-natal which is post-partum depression. The woman will also be educated on the resources that are important to having a successful pregnancy and stable post pregnancy.
Infant – Neonatal Abstinence Syndrome (NAS)	The woman will be educated thoroughly on the reasons for NAS along with the symptoms and the areas that NAS affects (autonomic, gastrointestinal and neurological systems). The woman will be educated on the assessments that are used in the NICU along with the scoring of the infants by the nursing staff and the neonatologist. The woman will be prepared of how she will be able to participate in the care of her infant while he or she is going through NAS. The education will also entail the pharmacology that assists the infants with NAS.

As the mother becomes educated on the four components of the Positive Direction Matrix the Positive Direction Model is introduced along with the concept that the woman is part of her treatment and the pregnancy outcome. The woman will utilize the Positive Direction Matrix in conjunction with the Positive Direction Model to create treatment goals to assist with staying on task and focusing on the health of her unborn child. The woman will begin to use a composition notebook to take notes and add educational information as it is distributed. The purpose of the woman using the composition notebook is for the woman to reflect on meetings as well as journal about her pregnancy.

As she journals and takes specific notes with guidance this will assist formulating and asking questions to her OB GYN or other medical providers involved with the prenatal treatment. The use of the notebook will also assist the woman to create goals and to be in control of her pre-natal health. The woman's ability to document in her own way will assist the mother to become self-reliant and motivated for treatment and a healthy infant. This "how to" Positive Direction Model is a self-directed program as well as a teaching tool that the mother is responsible for the infants outcome with the guidance of the navigator. Since the Positive Direction Model is self-directed the mothers take ownership for their pregnancy and the outcome. The model requires the mother does daily homework which entails researching and conferring with the medical professionals with the Navigator throughout the pregnancy. The Positive Direction Model is also creating independence along with building self-reliance, self-efficacy to begin the journey of motherhood.

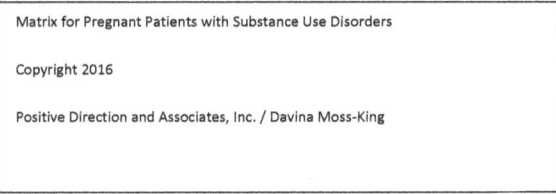

Matrix for Pregnant Patients with Substance Use Disorders

Copyright 2016

Positive Direction and Associates, Inc. / Davina Moss-King

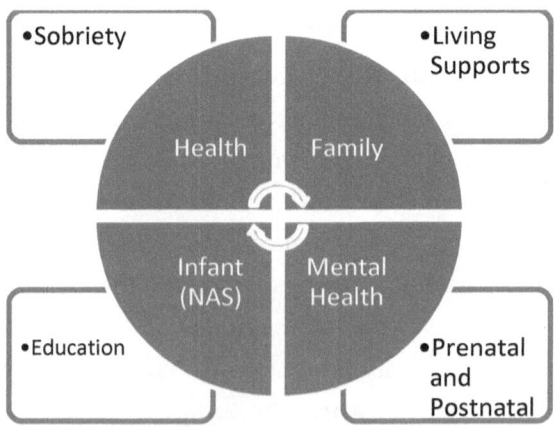

Figure 1

Case Study

Jennifer is a 25 year old that had surgery while in high school and was given a prescription of opioids for pain. Jennifer is a young woman that comes from a divorced family but has equal parental involvement. Jennifer has 1 older brother and 1 younger sister, both individuals had a history of alcohol use, but are in recovery now. Jennifer has expressed that there was an issue of alcohol use from her father along with cocaine use and that was the precipitant to the divorce of her parents. Jennifer states that her father is now in recovery but often struggles and relapses often. Jennifer states that she is very close to her father and is often upset when he relapses.

Jennifer confesses that she enjoys the feeling that she gets from opiates: feeling relaxed, numb and free. Jennifer stopped using the opiate medication but soon found herself purchasing from friends. Once she was not able to purchase from friends she was introduced to heroin. Jennifer began using heroin intranasal but soon began to use intravenously (IV) when she met her significant other who also uses heroin. Jennifer has been using now for approximately 5 years four to five bags per day IV and has attempted detoxification and rehabilitation twice. Each opportunity she had to attend substance use disorder outpatient she would not follow-through with her appointment. Jennifer stated that she would go back to her environment to live with her significant other and would begin to use again. Jennifer's significant other Douglas states that he has attempted to be clean but loves the drug too much and will not start to become clean until something major makes him.

Jennifer states that she used her heroin as she would normally, but she became violently ill and does not understand. Jennifer states that she has been vomiting daily and states nothing is helping. Jennifer admits that she has continued to use but is feeling "funny." Douglas suggests that she go to the emergency room for medical treatment. Jennifer goes to the emergency room complaining of nausea and admits that she is taking heroin on a regular basis. She states to the admission nurse that the nausea and vomiting is happening daily and would like to know what is wrong. The nurse forwards the information to the physician on staff and the doctor ordered a pregnancy test. The pregnancy test came back positive and the length of the pregnancy is unknown because Jennifer suffers from amenorrhea and is unsure of the last day of her menstrual cycle. Jennifer, however can remember the last time that she and Douglas were intimate and that was about 6 weeks ago.

The physician talks to Jennifer about prenatal care, opioid maintenance therapy and the medical consequences that the fetus will experience if the use of heroin is not handled properly. Jennifer was discharged from the emergency room and was given a list of recommendations that overwhelmed her and made her feel stressed. Jennifer stated that she knew she was wrong, but she used heroin to relax. Jennifer has continued to use despite the consequences discussed at the emergency room.

Jennifer made an appointment with an OBGYN because she wanted to know how many months she was and her options. Jennifer attended the OBGYN initial meeting and she has been informed that she is 8 weeks pregnant and she only missed one day when heroin was not used. Jennifer admitted that she has been using heroin at least four times a day and is afraid to stop because of the withdrawal. The OBGYN Dr. Ruttler explains to Jennifer that if she continues to use she will expose her infant to opioids and there could be consequences at birth that can require medical attention. Dr. Ruttler has given Jennifer the phone number of a prenatal navigator to assist with treatment for Jennifer and her unborn baby.

CHAPTER **2**

UNDERSTANDING OPIOID USE DISORDER

According to the American Society of Addiction Medicine (2015), "addiction is a primary, chronic disease of brain reward, motivation, memory and related circuitry. Dysfunction in these circuits leads to characteristic biological, psychological, social and spiritual manifestations. This is reflected in an individual pathologically pursuing reward and/or relief by substance use and other behaviors" (ASAM, 2015, pg. 13). In other words, an individual introduced to a substance can become addicted over time when he or she continues to use the substance to continuously achieve the same reward feeling. The health section of the matrix can be addressed by addiction counseling / substance use disorder counseling is conducted by a credentialed or licensed professional, usually in an office setting or in a rehabilitation facility. Substance use disorder counseling involves a professional teaching an individual coping skills to minimize or discontinue harmful substance use and help the individual understand the consequences of continued use. This credentialed professional could be a Licensed Mental Health Counselor that focuses on mental health diagnosis along with addiction, or a licensed / credentialed substance abuse counselor who focuses on substance abuse diagnosis. Professionals from other disciplines, like psychology, psychiatry, and social work, are also able to counsel individuals with a substance use disorder. These professionals are specifically trained in the area of substance abuse and alcoholism and are able to provide effective individual treatment.

At the juncture of the 21st century opioid dependence has become a public health problem nationally and internationally involving women has become an epidemic (Winklbaur, Kopf, Ebner, Jung, Thau and Fischer, 2008; Darnall, Stacey and Chu, 2012). Women have been prescribed opioid medications for pain and for various medical ailments more disproportionately than men and causing complications such as insomnia, and gastrointestinal medical issues to name a few. The most common use of opioid prescriptions for women is for chronic pain management where dependence can most likely occur. Other uses of opioids prescribed for women may be part of the pharmacological aftercare regimen following surgery, which could include but not limited to a cesarean section and / or hysterectomy (Darnall et. al., 2012). The most commonly prescribed medications are codeine, hydrocodone, and oxycodone not excluding the illicit drug heroin which some women may begin using after becoming addicted and the resources for prescriptions are no longer available.

Opioids are considered an analgesic and a pain inhibitor that can have physiological effects of the respiratory system. The respiratory system slows down when the opioid is ingested and crosses the blood barrier; euphoria begins and pain is dulled (Howard, 2003; Moss-King, 2009). The opioid can affect the brain function and the nervous system with physical effects such as nausea and sometimes vomiting and an itchy feeling on the skin which results from histamine(s) released from the opioid. Along with skin problems the digestive tract is compromised by the use of the opioid creating constipation and other digestive medical issues (Brezina, 2009). Women can suffer from secondary amenorrhea which means the menstrual cycle has been absent for approximately three months or more (Brezina, 2009). As a result, the woman may become pregnant and blindly continues using or abusing opioids which can be harmful to the mother and the fetus as well.

Some other adverse effects of opioid use: sedation, cough suppression, dry-mouth, and miosis. Since the opioid has a half-life of 24-36 hours women as well as men continue to use opioids to avoid withdrawal symptoms. Some symptoms of withdrawal are (Opioids.Net, 2014; Stevens, 2013):

Confusion
Hallucinations
Delirium
Urticarial vasculitis
Hypothermia
Bradycardia
Tachycardia
Orthostatic hypotension
Headache
Urinary retention
Muscle Rigidity
Myoclonus
Flushing or biliary spasm
Vomiting
Perfuse sweating
Perfuse shakiness

Withdrawal from opioids requires monitoring and medical managing at a facility or a hospital qualified to provide such sensitive intensive care (SAMHSA, 2009). A medically managed facility can be a hospital or an agency where detoxification takes place. An individual enters this type of treatment to cleanse the body safely avoiding any serious medical issues. Methadone or Suboxone medications are given during this medical procedure for approximately five days of slowly decreasing or tapering the dosage while monitoring the vital signs very closely. Although detoxification is highly recommended when a woman has a desire to be clean and sober, it is however, not recommended for pregnant women because of the harmful effects to the fetus (SAMHSA, 2008, 2009).

Pain medications have different effects on men than on women. Women between the ages of 25 and 54 are most likely prescribed opioid pain medications; and women between the ages of 45 and 54 are most likely to die from an overdose (CDC, 2013). The medical issues that will encourage a physician to prescribe opioids range from chronic pain to work injuries that has a negative effect on the woman's Quality of Life (QOL). Females in society have various roles from caretaker, spouse to provider of the family. Their roles are significant and enhance our communities, workplace and households. The main objective of the women when seeking medical intervention is to cease the pain and continue the activities without interruptions. For this reason physicians may prescribe opioid medications for a longer time in comparison to men. The duration and amount can and usually lead to dependence which is a trajectory because the QOL is now decreased and compromised. Women are often seen in emergency rooms for painful ailments such as migraine headaches, facial pain, abdominal pain, fibromyalgia along with back and neck pain (Harvard Health, 2012). Along with the pain, the woman may suffer from mental health issues, such as depression or possibly anxiety that will lead to an additional prescription of Selective Serotonin Re-Uptake Inhibitors (SSRI's) and tricyclics (Winklbaur, et. al, 2008).

Recently, there has been reports that opioid use and misuse has become a public health problem that infants are born exposed to opioids. The statistics from the Center for Disease Control and local as well as international neonatal intensive care units has brought awareness to various communities of the danger combination of opoid use / abuse and women. In July 2012 United States Senator Charles Schumer from New York State recommended that the United States Food and Drug Administration provide clear labels on all opioid medications highlighting the physiological effects for women (Schumer, July 2012). The epidemic has reached across cities and small towns along with stretching beyond race and ethnicity which has forced the medical community to do more research and to heighten awareness of maternal and infant mortality in relationship to opioid use disorders. Along with the heightened awareness there comes a need for more services for the women that are addicted and will prioritize treatment because of pregnancy. In 2016 President Barack Obama signed into legislation for more funds to be available for treatment and this will especially be beneficial for women. It is important to note that in some areas of the United States treatment is scarce or that women are fearful of being judged and will not seek treatment along with prenatal care.

Chapter 3 will introduce and explain in detail the Positive Direction Model and how its use will improve relationships between providers and pregnant women breaking the barriers for judgment and focusing on the health and well-being of the unborn child. The notebook will be introduced as part of the model as a support supplement for the mother.

CHAPTER **3**

POSITIVE DIRECTION MODEL

Taking into consideration the number of providers that are involved with the woman before pregnancy the providers only increase with pregnancy. There is, however, one consistent problem that will make a difference in the woman's pregnancy and her infant's first stages of life in utero is the communication of all providers. In this century and in the age of the digital world there is still a need for communication. It is imperative that each provider understands and is informed of the changes in the woman's health. If a woman has a substance use disorder provider he or she will be expected to contact the Opioid Maintenance Therapy (OMT) provider, however, now who will contact the OBGYN? This is an important question and there is an answer: a navigator that arranges, and communicates with all the providers in the network of the mother and her infant. The Positive Direction Model has the mother and the infant as the network center and the navigator connects all providers to the "network" and begin relationships that are conducive for the health and well- being of the mother and her infant (see figure 2). The navigator along with the OBGYN are on her first layer followed by the second layer of providers the OMT, behavioral health specialist, substance use disorder counselor and the pediatrician. The navigator is the "go-to" organizer and communicator for the providers and the mother. It is imperative that communication is strong especially in the area of medication management and other prescriptions even over the counter prescriptions. The navigator also works with the mom to empower her to become an advocate for herself and her child. Also since communication is continuous through the pregnancy it will encourage the mother to discuss any changes with a provider that she has an interaction. The navigator provides a journal for the mother to use daily. This journal is used to write summaries of the visits with her providers and also formulate questions. The journal can also be utilized as a communication tool to voice the concerns of the mother to the providers.

Positive Direction Model

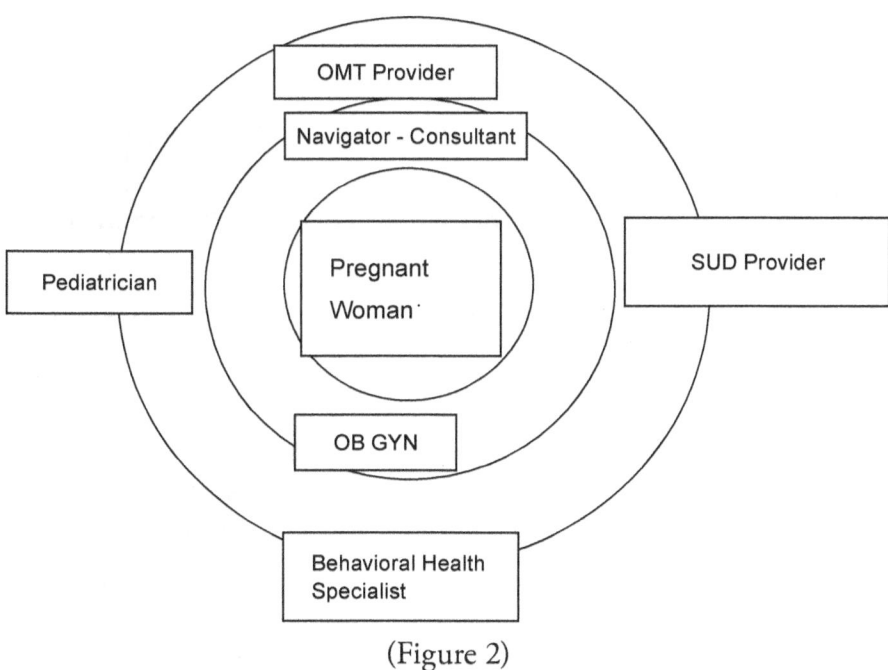

(Figure 2)

The purpose of the model is to integrate treatment for the progression of the patient along with the health of the mom and the health of the infant. The model navigator is the glue between the providers and the pregnant patient. The number one issue that is being addressed is the health and well-being of the infant.

✦ Jennifer feels very comfortable calling the navigator Gloria and sets up an appointment where Gloria discusses the Opioid Maintenance Replacement Therapy and also gives Jennifer a mental health assessment to identify any other issues related or unrelated to the substance use. Gloria then refers Jennifer to a Behavioral Health Specialist and also discusses the importance of mental health in relationship to the pregnancy. Gloria then relays all of this information to Dr. Ruttler; keeping the communication open between all health providers. Jennifer then begins to see Gloria bi-weekly. During the bi-weekly visit the two begin to work on a "workbook" that will be primarily for Jennifer and her baby. Gloria also invites Douglas to attend the sessions and be a participant in the bi-weekly sessions. Douglas states, "he will attend the biweekly meetings."

Jennifer begins to journal her experience and summarizes all the meetings for her and Douglas to review.

Navigator

The navigator is a professional that is working with the pregnant woman and can be referred by an OB GYN or might be an intricate part of a mental health or a substance use disorder clinic. The navigator will be the connecting glue between the mother –to – be and all of the providers connecting to the woman while she is pregnant. The navigator will be the coordinator of care and the organizer of the "notebook" to guide the woman through pregnancy and have her prepared enough for labor and delivery. The "notebook" will have the following table of contents: Section 1: demographics; Section 2: Treatment Plan; Section 3: Continuity of Care Providers; Section 4: Opioid Maintenance Therapy Letter of Confirmation; Section 5: My Birthing Plan; Section 6: Information for my Baby; Section 7: Discharge Plans; and finally,

Section 8: Ready to come home checklist. These sections will be gradually completed by the end of the pregnancy. The "notebook" in combination with the journal will empower the mother-to-be to ask questions, increase self-efficacy and be very prepared through the pregnancy to delivery. The mothers-to-be that have used the Positive Direction Model "notebook" and journal have had successful pregnancies where they were very involved with their pregnancy and became attached to their infants while pregnant. A mother that develops a relationship with her infant while pregnant will look forward to continuing the relationship afterbirth.

The continuation of the relationship forms a healthy bond and attachment that is healthy for the infant as well as the mother. A relationship with proper attachment is helpful for the mother to believe that she has the ability to care for and take care of her infant. This attachment is healthy for the infant to avoid Reactive Attachment Disorder (RAD).

Reactive Attachment Disorder

Reactive attachment disorder is a rare but serious condition in which an infant or young child doesn't establish healthy attachments with parents or caregivers. This is a condition found in children who may have received grossly negligent care and do not form a healthy emotional attachment with their primary caregivers -- usually their mothers -- before age 5. Attachment develops when a child is repeatedly soothed, comforted, and cared for, and when the caregiver consistently meets the child's needs. It is through attachment with a loving and protective caregiver that a young child learns to love and trust others, to become aware of others' feelings and needs, to regulate his or her emotions, and to develop healthy relationships and a positive self-image. The absence of emotional warmth during the first few years of life can negatively affect a child's entire future. RAD can affect every aspect of a child's life and development. There are two types of RAD: inhibited and disinhibited (Hornor, 2008).

Common Symptoms of Inhibited RAD Include

Women that are detached from their caregiver as an infant will have difficulty when she has her own children because the ability to be attached has never been felt or a learned behavior. As a woman that maybe in recovery and has been diagnosed with RAD this complicates the woman's ability to be an efficient parent. As an infant the woman may have been unresponsive or resistant to comforting by a foster parent or by anyone that had attempted to provide comfort. As an adult the woman would be excessively inhibited and unable to express their emotions.

Common Symptoms With Disinhibited RAD Include

Women with this type of RAD will have difficulty becoming familiar or selective in the choice of attachment figures as children and this carries on into adulthood when the woman becomes a caregiver. RAD occurs when attachment between the woman and her primary caregiver as a child or the woman and her present child. The lack of relationship bonding occurs or is interrupted due to grossly negligent care. This can occur for many reasons, including:

- Persistent disregard of the child's emotional needs for comfort, stimulation, and affection
- Persistent disregard of the child's basic physical needs
- Repeated changes of primary caregivers that prevent formation of stable attachments (for example, frequent changes in foster care)

There are various strategies for women that have been proven to be helpful for women in recovery. Statistics have shown that women who have appropriate coping mechanisms along with proper outlets will have lesser depression and have appropriate coping strategies.

Coping mechanisms have been an important part of a woman's recovery. The importance of having coping skills gives women an opportunity to have solutions to problems. The main reason that women relapse is because they lack solutions to the complex issues that arise in their daily lives. The coping mechanisms can be creating a notebook of various situations that may arise as triggers and then write various solutions to the specific situation. These solutions are known as coping mechanisms. The woman can review the solutions through role playing with the therapist and also with her support system. The more the woman engages with discussing her coping mechanisms the more automatic her responses will be to have a lesser chance to relapse.

The developing of coping mechanisms is important but also the need for support groups is also an important factor for women recovering from substance use disorders. Literature has stated that support from other women is a way to improve the self-efficacy and self-esteem for a recovery success. There are various support groups that are helpful to women in recovery such as post-partum depression group, women's group for addiction such as women for sobriety to name a few. There are also on-line chat rooms that are helpful for women who have very busy schedules and are not able to leave their homes to attend a meeting. The need for support groups brings on a comradery that allows women to understand they are not alone and will have support to bounce ideas off of others and also to encourage change. There are other groups that are useful such as book clubs and theatre clubs that assist the woman to learn to develop appropriate relationships and also relationships that do not revolve around substance use disorders and recovery. If the woman become involves in other groups it will assist her developing hobbies and also enhance her interests to do activities that do not involve the use of alcohol and or drugs. One of the main reasons some women have difficulty with returning to previous hobbies that were enjoyed is because the women state these hobbies were done under the influence. As a result, to return to these past hobbies will be trigger for relapse and an introduction for new hobbies or creative opportunities will need to be introduced by the therapist or the support system.

Finally, some women may be in need of a support systems such as domestic violence support group to give the women the confidence to have appropriate solutions to handle their situation without the use of alcohol or drugs as a coping mechanism. Women are in need of domestic violence support groups to assist the women to have proper guidance when they are attempting to make a decision to leave a significant other that is abusive. Statistics have shown that women that stay in abuse relationships usually continue in addiction. The women will stay in active addiction because it actually assists them with coping with their domestic violence situation. The purpose of the support group is to keep the women aware of their decisions and how it will impact their future or their children. The use of domestic violence court is also an important piece since it serves as a mediator for women in domestic violent situations and can also be used as a gait for safety.

The next support group that is important is a parent support group / classes. According to the program EPIC (Every Person Influences Children) groups and / or classes assist parents to learn alternative ways to discipline and also ideas to form a loving environment for children. Groups that educate and provide guidance of this type are necessary since the women may have a diagnosis of RAD and will benefit from learning alternative ways to parent for the success of their children. The need for parent groups is so important to give the women the support needed because the women will have an opportunity to discuss their struggles with other mothers. The need to balance family with the opportunity to stay clean and sober is very important and a worthwhile investment. Since there is an influx in children being referred to the department of social services – child protective services unit for children left unattended or not properly cared for, the support groups are essential to a positive home environment and recovery.

Responsibilities of the Navigator

The navigator is responsible to coordinate care for the woman. Besides organizing all appointments to include the providers from the Positive Direction Model the navigator will need to discuss possible inclusion of Child Protective Services (CPS). It is imperative that the navigator explains that the referral to CPS is under the policy and procedure and the discretion of the hospital / birthing center. The navigator will explain the importance of the OMT Provider letter which explains the prescribed medication along with the daily dosage. Since the OMT Provider letter and maybe the psychiatric provider letter states all medications that may pass the placenta and expose the infant these should be the only medications found in the infant's system. It is imperative that the navigator explains that if other substances are part of the toxicology report there maybe contact with Child Protective Services to investigate the safety and well-being of the infant.

Lastly, the navigator develops a relationship with the mother-to-be that allows the mother to speak freely and to become self-reliant. This independence becomes a microcosm from the intimate relationship with the navigator to a developing relationship with the infant.

Pregnant Woman

Pregnancy can be a rollercoaster and is difficult if going through all the stages alone. The mother becomes very independent if she is following the Positive Direction Model and soon becomes invested in her sobriety and treatment. The mother-to-be becomes excited about her progress and the success she is having with the pregnancy. The success can include but not limited to: developing appropriate sobriety strategies, creating a network of individuals that are invested in the pregnancy and the results, and lastly the infant becomes the motivating factor to continue progress.

The most difficult time is after the infant is born. The curiosity is heightened for the health of the infant and if neonatal abstinence syndrome will be a concern for the mother and her significant other and / or her family. At this point it is highly recommended that the mother returns to her "notebook" to review the information and has the confidence to ask more questions to be an involved party in her infant's treatment. Since the navigator has most likely referred the mother to various community groups while she was pregnant and the network will continue providing a support system post-partum.

The Positive Direction Model was developed a guide for mothers-to-be know the providers that are recommended to be involved with their pregnancy. Also the model was developed to encourage women to become invested in their pregnancy and the outcome of a healthy birth. Following the healthy birth it is recommended that the mother continues on the OMT and also mental health counseling if applicable to maintain the healthy environment created during the pregnancy.

Referral Process

This next section will take each provider and explain the role and the significance with the patient. The following individual providers will be discussed separately: OBGYN, OMT Provider, SUD Provider, Mental Health Provider, and Pediatrician.

Obstetrician Gynecologist

The OBGYN is a provider that will assist a woman through pregnancy and delivery. The woman is seen by the OB GYN at least every four weeks in the beginning; every other week and finally every week toward the end of the pregnancy. These appointments are of course depending on the medical condition of the mom and the possible medical condition of the fetus. The OBGYN has a relationship with the mom first hand because of the pregnancy. The OBGYN, however, has some concerns that the mom is a past user / current user of opiates. The following concerns arise when the OBGYN becomes aware of the mom's issues: toxemia, HIV, hepatitis C, miscarriages, infant mortality, still births, death of the mother during child birth, hypertension, and a small head circumference for the infant.

Since the OB GYN has many concerns regarding the woman that is pregnant and opioid dependent there is a need for mental stability and constant positive attitude.

Opioid Maintenance Therapy Provider

(OMT)

The Opioid Maintenance Therapy Provider is a physician that is trained in addiction along with the training sponsored by SAMHSA to administer suboxone and subutex also known as buprenorphine or subsolve. According to the Drug Addiction Treatment Act of 2000 (DATA 2000), physicians must complete an eight-hour training to qualify for a waiver to prescribe and dispense buprenorphine in an office setting (SAMHSA, 2016). The physicians that have been trained to dispense / administer the medication can be internal medicine physicians or other specialties. The specialty that would be helpful if the OB GYN was able to dispense the medication along with monitor the woman's pregnancy. Currently, nurse practitioners and physician assistants are able to attend the eight hour training to dispense the medication under the supervision of the physician. The OMT provider manages the dosage of the buprenorphine or suboxone for the length of the pregnancy. The navigator will have contact with the OMT during the pregnancy and in the third trimester the communication is imperative so that documentation can be given to the hospital along with the OB GYN. The OMT is an important factor for a successful pregnancy and delivery. The mother-to-be will use her journal to ask questions of the OMT related to the pregnancy and related to any side effects that may be experienced because of the medication that will be taken throughout the pregnancy. After delivery the OMT and the mother will review the medication dosage and the treatment plan for continuing or discontinuing the medication.

Behavioral Health Specialist

Behavioral Health counseling description is important aspect of the pregnancy being healthy from the beginning to delivery. There is a need to connect behavioral health with the OBGYN and the navigator may relay the mental health issues surrounding the pregnancy. It is important to understand that not all pregnancies are strategically planned. There is a need to connect the mental health to the pre and post natal treatment and in turn creates an environment that is conducive to the mother and the infant. The role of the behavioral health specialist is also to give education on post-partum depression and the solutions to handling the disorder proficiently with outside support. Outside support can consist of self-help support groups a close friend or family member to discuss many situations where self-doubt may interfere with the mother's ability to make decisions. The media has created a fantasy image of how a woman should experience their pregnancy and at times this could be a lonely and or depressing experience. Studies over the years have shown that women who experience depression prior to becoming pregnant will have a higher risk for experiencing depression while pregnant followed by post-partum depression. The behavioral health specialist's responsibility is to education the woman on the effects the mental health stability has on the pregnancy and the pregnancy experience. The mother may be experiencing negative feedback from family members, friends or other professionals. These judgmental verbal and non-verbal cues feed into society's stigma of women and addiction. There is a stigma especially for women that are pregnant and have a diagnosis of substance use disorder. The negative experiences lower the self-esteem and interferes with the woman's confidence to improve her health as well as her unborn child.

Through this process the behavioral health specialist is developing a trusting relationship with the mom and allows the mom to discuss the positive and negative aspects of her pregnancy that has been documented in her journal. Also this trusting relationship revolves around positive and effective communication where it becomes a microcosm for other relationships that are part of the Positive Direction Model.

The behavioral health specialist can administer assessments that will be important for the continued progress of the mother after birth. Such assessments are: The Beck Depression Inventory, The Edinburgh

Postnatal Depression Scale and The Maternal Lifestyle Post-Partum Questionnaire.

Beck Depression Inventory	20 questions that identify if the woman is mild, moderate or severely depressed.
Edinburgh Postnatal Depression Scale	Used to review the mother's emotions within a 7 day period.
Maternal Lifestyle Post-Partum Questionnaire	An assessment that asks indirect questions regarding the consumption of beverages other than milk or coffee and also identifies nutritious meals along with the lifestyle of the mother.

The Positive Direction Model can be successful because the navigator will communicate with the behavioral health specialist will communicate often with the OB GYN and or the staff to address any issues that arise during and even soon after the pregnancy. The behavioral health specialist must also work in unison with the navigator by providing reports after each visit and discussing the treatment plan to either continue the current goals or create new goals that will be conducive to the pregnancy and thereafter.

Since the mother may be on a Opioid Replacement Therapy it is salient that the substance use disorder counselor develop a healthy relationship with the navigator. This next section will discuss the role of the substance use disorder counselor and their role to enhance the woman's pregnancy experience by developing mental health coping skills to remain abstinent during and after pregnancy.

Substance Use Disorder Counseling

The role of the substance use disorder (SUD) counselor is to work with the woman and her motivations to staying sober during and after the pregnancy. The SUD counselor also creates treatment planning goals that will include but are not limited to coping skills, understanding the physiological and psychological effects of the drug on the woman as well as the physical effects on the fetus and even after-birth. The SUD counselor will spend and enormous amount of time discussing lifestyle changes that are conducive to recovery and to the well-being of the child. Such changes could include developing healthy relationships with non-users also redeveloping family relationships and child friendly activities.

The SUD counselor will also discuss with the emotional impact of motherhood in conjunction with relapse prevention strategies and coping effectively with stress from the new level of responsibilities. Discussing triggers is a vital part of counseling while the mother is pregnant. This strategy is especially necessary if a mother has more than one child in her care along with a newborn can be overwhelming. According to (Moss-King, 2013) stress is a trigger for individuals that are attempting to recover from opioid use and there needs to be more than one strategy for triggers that are discussed in the counseling session.

The SUD counselor is also affective by discussing sober activities that can be created while pregnant and then strategizes for activities post- partum. Along with these sober social activities the counselor should also discuss relaxation techniques that are appropriate without the use of opioids or other substances especially alcohol. This is the opportunity that the SUD counselor can give psycho-educational information on the changes in the hormone level afterbirth and the negative effect alcohol, opioids or other substances has on the mother and her ability to perform her daily activities.

The substance use disorder counselor's role is to identify the severity of the substance and to provide phases of treatment that can be completed through various counseling techniques such as motivational interviewing, cognitive behavioral therapy and reality therapy just to name a few. The counselor's role is to assist with brainstorming and developing coping mechanisms to help the mom pre and post-partum. Coping mechanisms can be relaxation techniques, exercise, alternatives to an unhealthy lifestyle to cope with stress and the newness of becoming a mother clean and sober.

Pediatrician

The pediatrician's role is the last part of the model that is salient to the continued success of the infant as he or she progresses through the developmental stage milestones. Prior to the birth it is highly recommended by the Positive Direction Model that the mother / parents begin to seek a pediatrician that will be an appropriate fit for their child. The definition of an appropriate fit / placement is a pediatrician that has experience with infants born exposed to opioids or other substances and diagnosed with neonatal abstinence syndrome. The pediatrician will also need the non-judgmental quality toward mothers in recovery or mothers that may be prescribed OMTs. The protocol within the model states that families should interview the pediatric practice with the guidance of the navigator. The mother / parents should have an opportunity to meet the physicians, nurse practitioners, physician assistants and nurses that will be involved with the infant's care. Some examples of questions:

(1) What is your practice's experience with neonatal abstinence syndrome infants?
(2) If I have questions / concerns regarding my infant what procedure is in place for me to contact your office during and off business hours?
(3) Does your practice communicate with the hospital staff before my infant is discharged regarding the infant's symptoms, medication management, length of stay in the hospital, assessments that were administered and the score results?

(4) How often are infants with neonatal abstinence syndrome seen by the pediatrician in your practice?

(5) Are there any developmental concerns for neonatal abstinence syndrome infants that I should be concerned with as my infant progresses through the developmental stages?

CHAPTER **4**

PREGNANCY

Women may discover that they are pregnant during the first three months (trimester) and may lack pre-natal care (Ornoy, 2002). There are a few reasons for lacking pre-natal care: (1) the woman is suffering from amenorrhea; (2) has been homeless and is lacking self-care; (3) in active addiction and participates in high risk behaviors continuously; or (4) lacks appropriate medical coverage. It is important for the woman to know the warning signs of a possible pregnancy: (1) complaining of nausea and not in active withdrawal; (2) tender breasts; (3) sensitive to unusual smells; and (4) extremely tired (Nilsson & Hamberger, 2004). Once these symptoms are observed immediate medical attention is warranted. Pregnant women actively using opioids causes obstetrics / gynecological complications such as toxemia, communal infections such as hepatitis C and HIV, low birth weight, still births, hypertension, excessive bleeding, miscarriages, small head circumference and early deliveries along with death of the mother and / or the fetus (Lin-Fu, 1969 and Jannson, Velez, & Harrow, 2009).

The woman may need to reach out to a community worker, a harm reduction counselor, a SUD counselor, or medical personnel which include the obstetrician / gynecologist, primary care physician, or a nurse practitioner when pregnancy is suspected. A pregnancy test may be administered and immediate focus is on the fetus and the safety and health of the mother. At this point the Matrix mentioned in Chapter 1 will begin to take shape for the success of the woman's health.

There are circumstances where a woman is under a physician's care for chronic pain and there is a suspicion of pregnancy, the physician will need to take immediate precautions. The physician will need to assess the medical condition of the woman prior to giving a new or refill prescription. The physician will also need to discuss the potential risk of dependence and the opioid substance being passed to the fetus causing complications during in utero development as well as congenital disabilities.

RECOMMENDED PHARMACOTHERAPY DURING PREGNANCY

Methadone and Suboxone are medications that can be used to avoid withdrawal in opioid dependent non - pregnant women as well as men.

According to SAMHSA 2008 suboxone was known to interfere with the skeletal development of the infant. However, within the past eight years there have been pregnant women that have taken suboxone through pregnancy and had success. There are more studies in the future to compare the opioid replacement therapies and the best practice for pregnant women. Therefore, it is important that the pregnant woman discuss their individual case with the Opioid Maintenance Treatment Provider to determine which medication will be administered.

This next section will discuss OMTs during pregnancy.

Methadone

Methadone has been the gold standard of treatment since the 1960's for maintenance and to avoid withdrawal during a medical managed detoxification. In addition to this, methadone has become the standard of treatment for pregnant women (SAMHSA, 2008). Methadone has been classified as a category C from the Food and Drug Administration since there is a lack of human studies. Although the FDA has concerns, mothers that were administered methadone properly and medically supervised were less likely to use other illicit drugs that would harm the fetus.

Once a medical professional has determined that methadone will be administered there is an induction as well as stabilization phases to the pharmacotherapy. The induction stage is to either continue the mother on the current methadone dose if the mother is currently taking methadone for maintenance at the time of pregnancy. If the mother has never taken methadone it is recommended by the Committee on Health Care for Underserved Women and the American Society of Addiction Medicine (2012) that the mother be admitted to the hospital for approximately 72 hours. During the hospital stay the opioid levels are assessed, the physical status of the mother along with the status of the pregnancy (SAMHSA, 2008; Jones et. al., 2012). The mother is observed for withdrawal symptoms and her weight, height and length of pregnancy is considered before administering the first methadone dosage.

During the last weeks of pregnancy the mother will be reassured that medication will continue with close monitoring after the delivery as well as an aftercare plan put in place for the safety of the mother and the child (Jones, Heil, Arria, Kaltenback, Martin, Coyle, Selby, Stine & Fischer, 2012).

There are medical reservations for mothers who are maintained on methadone maintenance during pregnancy. One main concern is most infants born from methadone maintenance mothers are exposed to the opioid resulting in acute withdrawal at least 3 hours to 12 days after birth. The acute withdrawal is called Neonatal Abstinence Syndrome (Franck, Harris, Soetenga, Amling, & Curley 2008). Although the infant is exposed, the positives of methadone outweigh the negatives expressed by physicians and researchers alike. The babies are born within the 36-38 week period, and born with average weight.

Methadone can be administered in a liquid form once per day in early pregnancy; however, as the pregnancy progresses 'split' dosing is recommended (SAMHSA, 2008). As the dose increases there are side effects for the mother according to Savage and Schofferman (1995) which are sleep disturbances, excess weight and fluid retention and an intolerance to pain during delivery where more medication is administered with caution and physician review.

Buprenorphine (Subutex)

The other option available to women is buprenorphine (Wesson & Smith, 2010).

Buprenorphine is a treatment that can be administered from an addiction trained physician (Moss-King, 2013). Various studies have illustrated that the administration of buprenorphine has lowered the use of other drugs and more mothers completed treatment as well as giving birth between 38-40 weeks (Wesson & Smith, 2010).

Studies have shown that the birth results are the same as mentioned earlier for methadone maintenance, however, the buprenorphine infants had less traces of the opioid in their system as was measured by their urine, umbilical cord testing and the meconium drug testing and they has less severe NAS symptoms (Soyka, 2013; Newman & Gevertz, 2011). As a result, the infants born exposed to buprenorphine spend less time in the Neonatal Intensive Care Unit and discharged from the hospital sooner than the methadone exposed infants.

CHAPTER **5**

FETAL DEVELOPMENT AND DELIVERY

Women that continue to take opioids such as heroin run the risk of overdose which the fetus will lose oxygen. The loss of oxygen can lead to the language and cognitive deficits which are recognized as the infant is developing. In the event that a pregnant woman does overdose it is recommended that Narcan can be administered to save the mother's life and gives oxygen to the unborn baby. There are other congenital birth defects that may occur according to the CDC (2013): (1) developmental delays, (2) spina bifida, (3) hydrocephaly, (4) glaucoma, (5) gastroschisis, (6) cleft palate, (7) congenital heart defects: (a) conoventricular septal defect, (b) tetralogy fallot and € pulmonary valve stenosis. According to Nilsson & Hamburger (2004) the heart and eyes are mainly affected because they are developing within the first three months of pregnancy. There is evidence that within the first few weeks of pregnancy the woman is unaware because of environmental issues such as homelessness or medical conditions such as amenorrhea which explains the lack of prenatal care. Also within the first few weeks of pregnancy the woman continues to use opioids and is unaware of the pregnancy hence forth the woman is exposing the fetus to the opioid along with other substances.

The first few weeks as the embryo develops approximately on the 22nd day the brain is unprotected and open exposing the brain to a variety of toxins from the substances administered by the mother; also on the 22nd day the heart begins beating at a very rapid pace (Nilsson

& Hamberger, 2004). The placenta has formed and is the nutritious connection between the uterus and the embryo. At this point the navigator will encourage a balanced diet and encourage abstinence of other substances except for the opioid maintenance therapy medication prescribed by the provider. The Positive Direction Model recommends the woman reviews her birth plan with the OMT and the OB GYN to discuss any concerns prior to delivery. Some concerns can be medication given during delivery and upon discharge. Upon the OB GYN reviewing the birth plan and the delivery, the woman can discuss the use of a doula or the use of a mid-wife during delivery. The role of a doula is to provide support to the mother and family during and after childbirth. The doula is a trained professional in the area of childbirth and the focus is to achieve a healthy birth that is a satisfying experience for the mother and support to the mother after the birth (DONA.org, 2017). The role of a mid-wife is to assist the woman during childbirth and minimizing technological interventions. The mid-wife is hands on during labor and delivery and will refer women to an obstetrician if needed (American Pregnancy.org, 2017).

Preparation for Delivery

The mother-to-be has been utilizing the previous months in her first and second trimester focusing on continuing abstinence, developing coping skills, and finally creating an atmosphere / environment that is conducive to welcoming her infant home. The Positive Direction Model utilizes the workbook along with the composition notebook to take notes, summarize sessions and identify any trouble spots of concern. Some areas of concern can be the care of the infant if diagnosed with NAS. The Positive Direction Model suggests that the mother – to – be takes a tour of the hospital that the delivery will take place and inquires on the form of treatment used for infants that are diagnosed with NAS. The inquiry will encourage communication between the mother and the medical staff and increases the mother's preparedness through education. During the third trimester the navigator will begin to focus on the birthing plan by completing the section in her workbook. The navigator will review if the mother – to – be has a plan for a Doula and or a Mid-Wife and who the support system will be during the labor and delivery process and also after birth. The navigator will assist the mother –to – be with packing an overnight bag to be ready. The navigator will review the items that are needed: (1) an overnight bag of her choice. (2) undergarments, (3) a breastfeeding bra, (4) night clothes, including a robe, skid-free socks or slippers, (5) hygiene hair products (dry shampoo) including a comb and brush, (6) change of clothes for the mother, (7) new outfit for the infant to be transported home, (8) a blanket for the infant, (9) the mother's Positive Direction Model Notebook which will be packed last on the way to the hospital.

During this preparation phase The Positive Direction Model highly recommends that he OMT provider completes a letter stating the dose of methadone or buprenorphine (subutex) and the dates that the mother – to- be has been a patient of the provider. This letter is given to the mother-to-be and she will laminate a copy of the letter. The laminated copy will go in the notebook the original copy will be given to the navigator. If the mother-to-be is involved with mental health counseling and there have been SSRI's taken during pregnancy the Positive Direction Model highly recommends a letter from the psychiatrist be written describing the medications prescribed. One week before delivery the navigator will fax both letters to the OB GYN, also a copy to the hospital nursing manager if there is an established relationship. The purpose of this is so that the hospital as well as the OB GYN are prepared and understand the medications that the infant may be exposed to in utero.

During the later months of the pregnancy the education regarding Neonatal Abstinence Syndrome is reviewed by the navigator and mother begins to prepare herself for any possibilities of difficulties after birth because of opioid use or Opioid Maintenance Therapy.

Neonatal Abstinence Syndrome Disorder

Neonatal Abstinence Syndrome Disorder consists of a group of symptoms as a result of opioid exposure to the unborn child. There are medications that can cause NAS symptoms: tobacco, benzodiazepines, SSRI's and opioids. The exposure can negatively affect the central nervous system. The areas affected: neurological, gastrointestinal and autonomic systems (Lin-Fu, 1969). Neurologically, the signs that the children experience after birth: irritability, staying awake for long periods of time and sleeping in short intervals, high pitch cries for long periods of time. The infant is not calmed easily and the infant may experience seizures, sneezing often, inability to suck along with stiff arms, legs and back along with the tarsal and other parts of the body having tremors with or without a moro reflex (Jannson, Choo, Velez, Harrow et al., 2009). The infant's gastrointestinal system is compromised and the result is vomiting, diarrhea followed by dehydration, inadequate weight gain caused by a lack of eating because of the inability to suck properly. Lastly, the autonomic system is affected and the medical staff will recognize this because the infant will have a fever, regulating the temperature is a constant struggle along with elevations in the respiration and the blood pressure will fluctuate often (Jansson, et. al, 2009). The infants that are diagnosed with Neonatal Abstinence Syndrome (NAS) are usually admitted to Neonatal Intensive Care Unit (NICU) where nurses and neonatologists take special care of the infants. The nurses and attending physicians will notice if the infant appears very uncomfortable and fidgeting and usually the infant is swaddled and may be given pharmacological solutions along with swaddling often and the use of "cuddlers" are helpful. Cuddlers are trained volunteers in the area of neonatal abstinence syndrome and are used to swaddle the infants and to hold the infant to encourage human contact which gives the infant comfort. The Positive Direction Model gives the mother information regarding the cuddler so this is not a surprise and the mother knows that she will have support through the night after the mother has been discharged. It is important to note as was discussed in the introduction, some infants diagnosed with NAS may stay in the hospital for more than 16 days and it is important for the mother to understand that her infant may need to stay in the hospital to maintain stability through pharmacology. The model also discusses the assessments that may be administered to the infant in the NICU. This next section will briefly describe the assessments used in the NICU for NAS.

NAS Assessments

Nurses and neonatologists and other medical staff are able to use the following assessments to identify the severity of NAS as well as using the assessments as a guide for the administration of medications under the discretion of the physician. The assessments are: (1) Finnegan Neonatal Abstinence Scoring System; (2) The Lipsitz Neonatal Drug – Withdrawal Scoring system; (3) The neonatal Withdrawal Inventory; (4) The Neonatal Narcotic Abstinence Scoring Index; (5) Withdrawal Assessment Tool – Version 1 (Jansson, et. al., 2009). The assessment that is most widely used in NICU's around the country is the Finnegan Scale. Since this scale may be administered on the mother's infant and with the model she will understand the scale and be more open to the results and to the treatment plans recommended by the nurse or the neonatologist.

Assessments

The Finnegan Neonatal Abstinence Scoring System is a 31 scale that will qualify for the severity of the NAS for the infant and the assessment can be administered every four hours. The neonatologist will assess the scores on the Finnegan and determine the treatment for the infant. The treatment can be pharmacological or non-pharmacological under the advisement of the neonatologist.

Although the Finnegan is widely used in the NICU to determine treatment there are other assessments that can be used in the NICU depending on the preference of the hospital management. This next section will briefly list other assessments that can be considered while the infant is in the NICU.

The Lipsitz Neonatal Drug Withdrawal Scoring system scale has eleven items and the scores are between 0 and 4. The Neonatal Withdrawal Inventory is an eight point checklist of seven NAS symptoms with four-point behavioral distress scale. The Neonatal Narcotic Withdrawal index is a scale that consists of six items that are related to NAS (Jansson, et.al., 2009). The Withdrawal Assessment Tool – 1 is an assessment to identify treatment for infants exposed to opioid and benzodiazepine and diagnosed with NAS (Franck, Harris, Soetenga, Amiling and Curley, 2008).

The Positive Direction Model suggests that the mother – to – be takes a tour of the hospital that the delivery will take place and inquires on the form of treatment used for infants that are diagnosed with NAS. The inquiry will encourage communication between the mother and the medical staff and increases the mother's preparedness through education. This education includes, but not limited to the protocol at delivery and the navigator at this time will explain the procedures and read information that is salient to delivery.

DELIVERY

This is an exciting yet very scary time for the mother and it can be even more difficult with the mixture of OMT and the feeling of being judged. The Positive Direction Model encourages self-efficacy because of the many months of preparing for the birth and understanding all of the components of NAS as much as possible. Upon entering the hospital the mother will share the OMT Provider letter which alerts the medical staff of OMT administered during pregnancy (Kashiwagi, Arlerttaz, Lauper, Zimmerman & Hebisch, 2005).

After birth the medical staff will assess the infant via a normal routine of scoring the infant by using the APGAR scores (Figure 3). These scores were developed by an anesthesiologist Virgina Apgar. Each letter represents the vital areas that need to be assessed immediately after birth to determine the health of the child as well as any medical procedures such as suctioning immediately after birth (Nilsson & Hamberger, 20004).

A = Appearance
P = Pulse
G = Grimace
A = Activity
R = Respiratory

(Figure 3)

The scores in each evaluation area range from 0-2; 0 being the lowest and 2 being the highest. The delivery attendant is responsible for observing the infant and relaying the score to the attending physician. Since there are five assessing areas the overall highest score is 10. The average score is 8-10 which means the infant does not need immediate attention; however, if the score is below 8 each low area is identified and medical procedures bein. The APGAR is performed at one and five minutes following the birth the two scores are compared to identify an increase or decrease in the overall score. If the score from five minutes does not show improvement then a third assessment of the APGAR is administered at ten minutes and the baby is assessed for a possible medical assessment and transferred to the neonatal intensive Care Unit (NICU).

Infants that are presenting with acute NAS may have an overall score below 8; however, there have been instances where the infant scores within normal range on the APGAR but within a few hours their health begins to deteriorate and NAS symptoms appear (Nilsson & Hamberger, 2004). According to Blandthorn, Forster & Love, 2011, there have been comparison studies that show there are no significant differences in the APGAR scores following the birth of the infants exposed to buprenorphine and methadone. With this information in mind the mother-to-be understands the reason the NAS Assessments become important to understand and the communication with the medical professionals becomes vital.

As part of the Positive Direction Model the navigator explains the mother's role with her infant after birth if diagnosed with NAS. One of the recommendations by the American Academy of Pediatrics (2012) is breastfeeding under the advisement of the neonatal medical team. The American Academy of Pediatrics also express that if the mother does not have health issues that may compromise the health of the infant breastfeeding is highly recommended.

BREASTFEEDING

As discussed earlier the third trimester with the Positive Direction Model navigator is focusing on the mother connecting with her infant and putting various structures in place for the mother to be successful. Breastfeeding is one of the areas that are reviewed in detail. The benefit of breastfeeding infants diagnosed with NAS is that it brings comfort and bonding between the mother and the infant and helps the infant. According to Balain and Johnson (2014) there is evidence to support that breastfeeding will assist to manage the NAS symptoms and possibly prevent NAS symptoms from becoming unmanageable. There is evidence that states that women that were involved with addiction activities have a low rate of engaging with breastfeeding. There may also be women that were involved with domestic violence whereas the breastfeeding is not an option because of damage or scarring on the breast. These feelings are translated to shameful and then the woman may not be interested in breastfeeding in private or in public. The navigator will address these emotions that are interfering with the woman's curiosity and the desire to connect with her infant by the breastfeeding mechanism.

The navigator will take into consideration the new mother has a list of concerns for beginning motherhood. The woman has may lack the confidence to breastfeed and she may not have the proper supports that will allow her the opportunity to actually embrace breastfeeding. At this point the navigator may refer the mother to a lactation consultant before she enters into the hospital. Meeting with the lactation consultant will ease the fears and minimize the list of uncertainties revolving breastfeeding. The Positive Direction Model highly recommends that the navigator discusses the research by Busch, Logan and Wilkinson (2014) where they created a Tri-Core Model from their extensive research for women that required support for breastfeeding. The Tri-Core Model is from Busch's 2013 research and the components are self-efficacy, mother and baby, lactation support and lactation education. This model has been very helpful for the mothers to be encouraged to breastfeed, meet their challenges and develop appropriate strategies to overcome barriers.

Positive Outcomes for Breastfeeding

Breastfeeding protects the infant, benefits the health of the mother and also is beneficial to promote bonding through skin to skin contact. The benefit of the mother breastfeeding her NAS infant immediately is that the newborn is feed the colostrum. Colostrum is a created in the body during pregnancy and immediately after birth. The colostrum is rich in nutrients and antibodies. Colostrum is also healthy for the infant's digestive system (Women's Health.gov, 2016). As mentioned earlier the infant diagnosed with NAS has concerns with the gastrointestinal system and breastfeeding will be gentle to the infant's digestive system which will minimize diarrhea and irritability. Breastfeeding also benefits the infant in the following areas: asthma, childhood leukemia, childhood obesity, ear infections, eczema, diarrhea and vomiting, lower respiratory infections, sudden infant death syndrome (SIDS), and type 2 diabetes just to name a few. The navigator will also link the mother to breastfeeding resources that are in their community along with resources on line and possibly a baby café. Baby café is a drop in center for mothers that are breastfeeding to find support, and meet other mothers that they can develop healthy relationships with through the breastfeeding process. At this café nutritious meals can be discussed and also fruit and vegetable platters can be distributed for the mothers along with informational pamphlets for other forms of support (thebabycafe. org, 2017).

Lastly, there are very useful APPs that will be very helpful for mothers to understand medications that can interfere with the breast-milk. The navigator will assist the mother-to-be with downloading an APP and this will also give support to embrace breastfeeding.

The combination of the navigator giving the information about the benefits of breastfeeding and setting the mother up with supports such as a lactation consultant and education, written resources available on the internet and android apps along with the baby cafés prior to the delivery date and admission to the hospital the woman will have the confidence to follow through breastfeeding after the birth of the infant.

The next chapter will discuss the last section of the Positive Direction Model and the last section of notebook which are the discharge plan for the infant and the follow through with medical appointments for the infant.

CHAPTER **6**

DISCHARGE PLANS

Since most infants are in the NICU ranging from four days to approximately 16 days or more there needs to be an appropriate address for the infant to reside after discharge (Harper, Solish, Purow, Sand, Panepinto, 1974). Identifying the residence and assisting with important items such as a crib, clothing, diapers, formula, just to name a few is the responsibility of the navigator. The navigator will also assist with following through with the discharge plans created by the hospital staff. The discharge plan should include a local pediatrician that is engaging and non-judgmental. It is the recommendation of the Positive Direction Model that the pediatrician is chosen before the birth of the infant as discussed in chapter three along with the list of possible interview questions that were also discussed in chapter three.

The mother or the caregiver will need to understand the care of the infant especially if he or she was born with congenital defects that could compromise the daily caretaking. It is appropriate that a nurse be involved and may give education to the mother / parents / caregiver on the correct protocol to take care of the infant properly. An infant could be diagnosed with glaucoma and the discharge plan would include the navigator helping with transporting or setting up appointments The appointments would be with an optometrist to monitor the progress of the disease. At this point the mother will include the discharge plans and the treatment plan for the infant in her "notebook" and begin to journal any concerns to discuss with the pediatrician or the specialist. The navigator will not only focus on the infant, but will discuss the importance of the environment where the infant will live. It is salient that the environment is calm and drug free.

Many studies have shown that mothers that were involved with alcohol and or drugs during and prior to their pregnancy were involved with a domestic violence situation (Wilson, McCreary, Kean, Baxter, 1979). Earlier it was discussed that the infant was exposed to opioids in utero. Now that the infant is discharged to home or to a new environment outside the hospital the exposure could be the parent in the home actively using in the presence of the infant. This exposure could lead to more violence and impede the child's development, especially language (Ornoy, 2002). Drug exposure could be linked to poor nutrition, neglect, emotional instability such as Reactive Attachment Disorder along with environment instability (DeCristofaro, & LaGamma, 1995). There is medical evidence that opioid exposure can affect motor coordination which includes fine and gross coordination along with cognitive delays. These cognitive delays later affect the child as a toddler with respect to short / poor attention spans, hyperactivity, learning disabilities, inadequate balance delayed speech and language development (DeCristofaro & LaGamma, 1995; Ornoy, 2002).

In the research study by Konijnenberg and Melinder (2012) researching OMT mothers they discovered that mirror neuron system (MNS) is affected. The MNS is a neural circuit that involves understanding cues and understanding social interaction. The main area affected was visual input which made watching another person and or learning from another person by visual cues for any length of time difficult. The results of this study gives a validation for hyperactivity and short attention span while toddlers were in a structured environment such as a pre-school classroom a constant challenge (Konijnenberg & Melinder, 2012).

It is recommended in the literature to follow-up with a pediatrician discussing the milestones in the preschool age. The mothers can also add apps on their mobile devices regarding the developmental stages of their children in comparison to the norms of other children in the same age range. Language delay is significant and assessments can be administered by age 2 by a speech language pathologist. According to the results early intervention plans are created to involve the parent / care giver, speech language pathologist and there could be an occupational therapist involved along with the pediatrician (Robertson & Weismer, 1999). Children that need this type of treatment team approach are referred to Early Intervention Services either by the pediatrician, the navigator or the Child Protective Services Worker. The early intervention services start with an assessment and then a plan is created with the necessary medical and therapeutic professionals to enhance the infant's educational and social life. This type of intervention can begin during infancy until age three. Usually at age three it is recommended that a child begins pre-school / universal pre-school for a half of day or an entire day. If there is a need for early intervention services to continue while the child is in pre-school there is a referral to the Committee on Special Education to begin the process of an Individualized Education Plan (IEP). The IEP can include the same specialized services as well as other services in the classroom that will enhance the child's academic opportunities. Most importantly, the family may require extra wrap around services that may not be a part of the IEP but are significant enough to create a healthy environment that encourages learning. If the mother takes the opportunity to use the Positive Direction Model efficiently then the mother and the infant are on a path of success and are able to create a positive environment.

What next?

Now that all levels of the Positive Direction (PD) model is explained and we have a clear understanding of neonatal abstinence syndrome and all of the components that create a healthy pregnancy for the pregnant mom let's look at the participants involvement.

"People do not remember what you said but they remember how you made them feel."

(Maya Angelou)

Individuals that are pregnant and have opioid use disorder have received stigma over many years. However, with the new epidemic the stigma has become even stronger. The individuals already feel under-empowered and judged. The purpose of the model is to increase self-esteem, increase self – efficacy and create empowerment. This model will provide the mom/dad and family with appropriate documentation so that their infant can be born healthy. The parents learn to supply appropriate documentation by keeping a simple cost effective composition notebook and documenting any issues or concerns regarding care or medication management. This method is done to increase the self-efficacy it is vital that the counselor use motivational interviewing to give the patient the opportunity to talk and enhance their life skills. The values of the lifestyle changes are vital to a healthy environment. It is vital that the mom begins to feel that she is going in a positive direction for her life as well as her infant.

The women are also able to complete a workbook that is provided by the Positive Direction Model to be of assistance for the providers and the navigator for effective treatment. The workbook consists of a birthing plan, information from the OMT provider, discharge plans, breastfeeding information, and lastly information regarding neonatal abstinence syndrome. A sample of the workbook is provided in Appendix A.

CONCLUSION

The epidemic of opioid use involving pregnant women is an epidemic that has reached across the United States and abroad. This epidemic is affecting the nation's future. Infants that suffer from NAS is due to exposure to opioids whether from Opioid Maintenance Treatment medications or from other opioid medications deserve to have an opportunity for a bright future. Since the results are so threatening from immortality to life-time congenital diseases because of loss of oxygen in the event the mother overdoses; other results include learning disabilities, behavior problems and cognitive deficits that impact language it has become necessary that every aspect of opioid medication is explained thoroughly especially to women. Through research, education and prevention and the correct supports in place from medical and academic community this epidemic will be managed properly. The mothers-to-be will be informed and will feel a part of their substance use disorder counseling and the OB GYN appointments.

The use of the Positive Direction Model along with the "notebook" in conjunction with the journal with the guidance of the navigator the women will be educated on the use of opioids and the exposure to the fetus. Allowing the women to have intensive services where she takes ownership of her treatment and the future of her infant. The use of the journal and writing treatment planning goals is insightful and powerful to encourage women to be motivated to continue sobriety during the pregnancy and after delivery. The Positive Direction Model can lead to increasing self-efficacy, raising her self-esteem and empowering the mother-to-be to make healthy decisions. This model assists the women to be educated about their health, utilize the resources and create coping mechanisms while pregnant and then continue these mechanisms after birth. The pride that the mother-to-be has for being able to have control over the birth of their infant is a gratifying experience for the navigator and all the professions involved in the mother's health care. It is with much hope that the Positive Direction Model can be used to assist women that are going through the process of recovery and are pregnant be successful and deliver healthy infants that are our future leaders.

REFERENCES

American Academy of Pediatric Committee on Drugs (2012). Neonatal drug Withdrawal. *Pediatrics*: 129: e540

American College of Obstetrician and Gynecologists Women's Health Care Physicians (May 2012). Committee on Health Care for Underserved Women and the American Society of Addiction Medicine. Opioid Abuse, dependence and addiction in pregnancy, Number 524, 1-7.

AmericanPregnancy.org (2017).

Balain, M. & Johnson, K. (2014). Neonatal abstinence syndrome: the role of breastfeeding. *Infant,* Volume 10 (1); pgs. 9-13.

Blandthorn, J., Forster, DA & Love, V. (2011). Neonatal and maternal outcomes Following maternal use of buprenorphine or methadone during pregnancy Findings of retrospective audit. Women Birth, 24(1): 32-39.

Busch, D., Logan, K., Wilkinson, A. (2014). Clinical practice breastfeeding recommendation for primary care: applying a tri-core breastfeeding conceptual model. Journal of Pediatric Health Care, 28 (6), p. 486-497.

Center for Disease Control and Prevention. National Center for Injury Prevention And control, Division of Unintentional Injury Prevention (July 2013). Prescription painkiller overdoses: a growing epidemic, especially among Women.

Center for Disease Control and Prevention (July 2013). National Center on Birth Defects and Developmental Disabilities. Key findings: maternal Treatment with opioid analgesics and risk for birth defects. Atlanta, GA.

Center for Disease Control and Prevention (2012). Infant mortality statistics from The 2008 period linked birth / infant death set. National vital statistics Reports. Volume 60 (5). Hyatttsville, MD.

Cleary, BJ., Donnelly, J., Strawbridge, Jl, Gallagher, PJ., Fahey, T., Clarke, M., & Murphy, DJ. (2010). Methadone dose and neonatal abstinence syndrome – Systematic review and meta-analysis. *Addiction, 105*, 2071-2084.

DeCristofaro, JD., & LaGamma, EF. (1995). Prenatal exposure to opiates. *Mental Retardation and Developmental Disabilities:* 1: 177-182.

DONA.org (2017)

Franck, LS., Harris, SK., Soetenga, DJ., Amiling, JK & Curley, MAQ (2008). The withdrawal assessment tool – version 1 (WAT -1): an assessment Instrument for monitoring opioid and benzodiazepine withdrawal symptoms In pediatric patients. *Pediatric Critical Care Medicine.* November. Vol. 9 (6): 573-580.

Hall, E.S., Isemann, B.T., Wexelblatt, S.L., Meinzen-Derr, J., Wiles, J.R., Harvey, S., & Akinbi, H.I. (March 2016). A cohort comparison of buprenorphine versus methadone treatment for neonatal abstinence syndrome. *Journal of Pediatrics (170)*, 39-44.

Hornor, G. (2008). Reactive attachment disorder. Journal of Pediatric Health Care, 22(4), p. 234-239.

Jansson, L., Choo, R., Velez, ML, Harrow, C., Schroeder, JR., Shakeleya, D., & Huestis, MA. (2008). Methadone Maintenance and breastfeeding in The neonatal period. *Official Journal of the American Academy of Pediatrics, 121(1),* 106-114.

Jones, H.E., & Fiedler, A. (November, 2015). Neonatal abstinence syndrome: Historical perspective, current focus, future directions. *Preventive Medicine (80),* 12-17.

March of dimes (Retrieved October 2015). http://www.marchofdimes. org/baby/neonatal-abstinence-syndrome-(nas).aspx#

Moss-King (2009) Unresolved Grief and Loss Issues Related to Heroin Recovery. Vom Verlag: Germany

Moss-King, D. (October 2015). Neonatal Abstinence Syndrome : Effects on our future. *Western New York Family Magazine.*

Moss-King, D. (2014). Management of opioid dependency during pregnancy. http://www.netce.com/coursecontent.php?courseid=1138

Moss-King, D. (2013). Individual Treatment pp. 188-201. Substance Abuse Counseling: Theory and practice: 5th Edition. Editors Stevens, P. and Smith, R. Pearson: New York, NY.

National Institutes of Health (2015). About LactMed. Retrieved from http://toxnet.nlm.nih.gov/newtoxnet/lactmed.htm

Opioids.net (2014). Opioids: pain management, addiction, treatment, effects And information. Retrieved February 18, 2014.

Ornoy, A. (2002). The impact of intrauterine exposure versus postnatal Environment in neurodevelopmental toxicity: long term neurobehavioral Studies in children at risk for developmental disorders. *Toxicology Letters:* 140-141: 171-181.

Robertson, SB., & Weismer, SE. (1999). Effects of linguistic and social skills in Toddlers with delayed language development. *Journal of Speech, Language And Hearing Research, 42*: 1234-1248.

Soyka, M. (2013). Buprenorphine use in pregnant opioid users: a critical review. *CNS Drugs, 27*: 653 – 662.

Substance Abuse and Mental Health Services Administration (July 2016). Buprenorphine Training for Physcians.

Substance Abuse and Mental Health Services Administration. Center for Substance Abuse Treatment (2009). Detoxification and Substance Abuse Treatment Training Manual.

Substance Abuse and Mental Health Services Administration: A Treatment Improved Protocol (TIP) 43 November 2008. Medication – assisted Treatment for opioid addiction during pregnancy. Chapter 13.

Thebabycafe.org (2017)

Tierney, S. (2013). Identifying neonatal abstinence syndrome (NAS) and Treatment Guidelines. University of Iowa Children's Hospital.

Wilson, GS., McCreary, R., Kean, J., & Baxter, JC. (1979). The development of Preschool children of heroin – addicted mothers: a controlled study. *Pediatrics, 63(1)*, p. 135-141.

www.womenshealth.org (2016). The benefits of breastfeeding.

Copyright 2016 – Positive Direction and Associates, Inc.

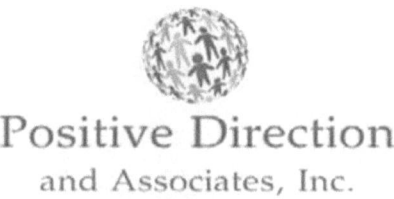

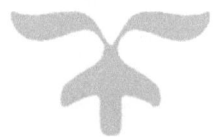

Davina Moss-King, Ph.D., CRC, CASAC, NCC
Consultant
Positive Direction and Associates, Inc.
Telephone #
Fax #

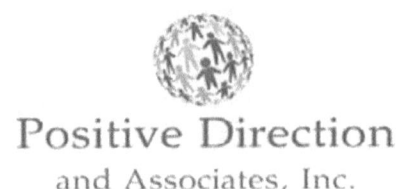

Positive Direction
and Associates, Inc.

This notebook belongs to

_____

Birthing Plan

TABLE OF CONTENTS

- Demographics
- Treatment Plan
- Continuity of Care Providers
- OMT Letter
- My Birthing Plan
- Information for my baby
- Discharge Plans
- Ready to come home checklist

✚ DEMOGRAPHICS

Name: _____

Address: _____

Phone #: _____

Emergency Phone #: _____

Medical Information: _____

Insurance Card Number for Mom and baby:_____
_____

OBGYN Information: _____

OMT Physician: _____

Pediatrician Information: _____

Other Agencies (Case Manager) Information:_____
_____

Medical Complications: _____

Medications taken during pregnancy: _____
_____

MY TREATMENT PLAN (PRE & POST PREGNANCY)

Client Name: Counselor Name:

Date	Problem Statement

Goals

Criteria	Objectives
	What will the client say or do? Under what circumstances? How often will he/she say or do this?

Interventions	Service Codes	Target Date	Resolution Date
What will the counselor/staff do to assist client? Under what circumstances?			

Participation in Treatment Planning Process

Participation by Others in the Treatment Planning Process

Client Signature/Date
Counselor Signature/Date

Place OBGYN Business Card Here	Place Positive Direction and Associates, Inc. Business card here
Place OMT Physician card here	Place outside agency business card here
Place outside agency business card here	Place Pediatrician business card here

SAMPLE

Provider Name
Provider Address
Provider City, State - Zip Code

Patient Name

To Whom It May Concern:

Patient Name is prescribed Xmg of _____
under the care of Provider's Name(s) since start date of admission
into the OMT Program. The medication is administered number
of times daily.

Please contact our office if you have any questions / concerns
Provider's contact information.

Provider's Signature

Important: Be aware if you are able to take your OMT medication
bottle with you to the hospital or if your OMT medication will be
"ordered" at the hospital for your daily dose.

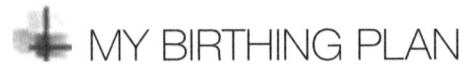# MY BIRTHING PLAN

| Name: |
| Due Date: |
| Labor Partners: |
| My Doula is: |

For My Labor I prefer:
____ Dim Light
____ Music
____ Silence
____ My own clothing and bedding

Mobility Pre-Labor
____ I would like to walk, safely change body positions
____ I would like to stay in bed except for using the bathroom
____ I would like an epidural and understand I may be confined to the hospital bed and will most likely have an urinary catheter

My nourishment and hydration
____ I prefer to eat light snacks and drink clear fluids if allowed
____ I am agreeable to have an IV for hydration
____ I am agreeable to discuss hydration with the hospital and follow the hospital's recommendation(s)

My fetal monitoring preferences

____ I agree to follow the hospital procedures and recommendation(s) for monitoring my baby before birth

____ I would like as much monitoring of my baby as possible

___ I prefer fetal monitoring while in bed

Birth Process:

____ The following people can-not be in the labor room with me:

1.

2.

3.

____ The following people are allowed to be in the labor and delivery room with me:

1.

2.

____ I would like to hold my baby immediately afterbirth and breastfeed as soon as possible with the help of the labor and delivery staff

____ I would like to have _____ involved with cutting the umbilical cord

____ I would like more information on storing the umbilical cord

____ I will discuss circumcision with the hospital staff if my baby is a boy

____ I would like all routine evaluations performed

____ I will be breastfeeding

____ I will be feeding via formula

____ I prefer to be in the room with my baby

My Cesarean Plan

____ The following people can-not be in the operating room with me for the cesarean section

1.
2.
3.

____ The following people can be in the operating room with me for the cesarean section

1.
2.

____ I would prefer the surgeon describe the surgery in detail "in real time"

____ I would prefer a spinal

____ I would prefer an epidural

____ I would like to have skin – to – skin contact with my baby after birth (cheek - to – cheek) if possible

____ I would like to release one arm to hold my baby after the surgery

____ I would prefer to breastfeed while in the recovery room

____ I would prefer to formula feed

____ I agree to all of the routine evaluations to be performed

INFORMATION / EDUCATION FOR MY BABY AT RISK FOR NEONATAL ABSTINENCE SYNDROME

1. **What is Neonatal Abstinence Syndrome?**

   Neonatal Abstinence Syndrome (NAS) is also called withdrawal symptoms that infants experience as a result of exposure to opioids or other drugs while the mother was pregnant. NAS may also appear if the mother used / prescribed methadone, subutex (buprenorphine), and even nicotine. The infant is treated in the Neonatal Intensive care Unit (NICU) and a neonatologist along with other medical staff will keep you informed of your baby's progress. Below are medications that may be a cause of NAS along with the systems affected.

Medications

Prescription Medication	Non-prescribed	Illegal drugs
Morphine Fentanyl Methadone Subutex Methadone Including any opioid medication SSRI	Nicotine	Heroin Cocaine (crack)

Systems Affected

Neurological	Gastrointestinal	Autonomic System
Irritability	Vomiting	Fever

Staying awake for long periods	Diarrhea	Inability to regulate temperature
Sleeping in short intervals	Dehydration	Elevations in respiration
High pitch cries for extended periods of time	Inadequate weight gain because of inability to suck	Fluctuation of blood pressure
Not calmed easily		
Possible seizures		
Sneezing often		
Stiff arms, legs and back, tarsal		
Tremors		

2. **What is an APGAR Score?**

   The APGAR score is the first evaluation given to your baby. The five sections are scored between 0 and 2. The medical personnel in the labor and delivery room *may* discuss your baby's score.

A	Appearance Skin Color
P	Pulse (Heart Rate)
G	Grimace Response (Reflexes)
A	Activity (Muscle Tone)
R	Respiration (Breathing Rate and Effort)

3. **What are some of the evaluations that could be used and what do they mean to me and my baby? Scores will determine if medication will be administered to the infant.**

*The Finnegan Neonatal Abstinence Scoring System
The Lipsitz Neonatal Drug – Withdrawal Scoring System
The Neonatal Withdrawal Inventory
The Neonatal Narcotic Withdrawal Index

*Most often used in NICUs (See Appendix A for an example of the Finnegan by permission of the Iowa Hospital

4. **How long does my baby stay in the hospital?**
   Your baby will be evaluated by a neonatologist and the discharge plans will be discussed in detail with you and family members.

5. **May I breast feed?**
   Breast feeding is highly recommended and a lactaid consultant from the hospital may visit with you to discuss recommendations.

6. **If I go home first and my baby stays how will I visit?**
   Most hospitals welcome you to visit and feed your baby according to the hospital's policy and procedures. It is highly recommended that there is continued contact with the baby until discharge.

7. **What happens when I get home with my baby?**
   You will be given a discharge sheet with a set of instructions as well as any necessary precautions that need to be taken. It is highly recommended that the baby receive lots of love and affection to build the attachment bond in the early years.
   Watch your baby's cues and body language!
   Your baby will give signs or cues that let you know what he or she likes, and what makes him or her uncomfortable. Learning to read your baby's "body language" will make you feel more *confident*.

Discharge Plan:

1. OBGYN Visit after Discharge:
2. Visiting Nurses Association Phone Number and visit dates
3. Following up with the OMT Appointment Date:
4. Pediatrician and Appointment:
5. Schedule to be made for the home: Feeding time(s):   Bathing time: Nap time(s):   Connection(s) Time with my baby:

I will attach my discharge papers here:

AM I (WE) READY FOR MY (OUR) BABY TO COME HOME?
MY (OUR) CHECK LIST

1. Do I (we) have a car seat?	
2. Do I (we) have a crib / bassinet?	
3. Do I (we) have sensitive skin products for my (our) baby i.e. wipes, diapers etc.	
4. Do I (we) have formula for sensitive digestive systems	
5. Do I (we) have a smoke free car and environment for the baby	
6. Did I (we) make an appointment with the pediatrician?	
7. Do I (we) know the warning signs to watch for if my baby gets ill and the precautions to take?	

www.ingramcontent.com/pod-product-compliance
Lightning Source LLC
Chambersburg PA
CBHW021018180526
45163CB00005B/2015